C.G. Walker

The Oceanic Mind

an Accidental Journey
via Bipolar Disorder
through to the Other Side

ISBN: 098808290X
ISBN 13: 9780988082908

Contents

Forward

THE OCEANIC MIND IS A MEMOIR that has truly been earned by its author. The writing is charming, intriguing, and riveting in a way that is completely authentic. Yet the achievement of this book goes further, perhaps because, though gifted, the author is not a professional writer. Somehow he manages to convey a living sense of what might be called "bipolar subjectivity" or "manic-depressive consciousness." Even as a clinician, I learned something new about those burdened with this diagnosis.

The author seems to be exquisitely aware of his freedom to play with the reader's doubts and fears in order to bring forth in language and story-telling the shifting state of mind that has plagued him for a lifetime. One is sometimes not sure whether in the telling he is naively caught up in a bipolar current of "delusion," or whether he is being "tongue in cheek." This capacity to sustain an atmosphere of ironic but also agonizing ambiguity hooks us directly into the bipolar experience: for example, the sometimes exhilarating but often frightening and/or depressing episodes of acute uncertainty about whether to trust one's own thought process; the intense anxiety of being simultaneously a critical observer and a compulsive participant in multiple and incompatible mental processes (a predicament that most of us are spared by filters that bipolars seem to lack).

There is no skirting here of the manic-depressive cycle and the existential precariousness of disrupted personal and work relationships. Yet at the same time, the intensifying effect of bipolar consciousness seems to create a potential for deeply reassuring experiences of convergence, in which the author may be tapping into mysterious currents of unconscious communication, connecting with agencies and energies that are strangely distributed in our environment.

The result is a compelling journey of the embodied mind, a paradoxical history of suffering that is "recollected in tranquility" (Wordsworth), conveying a sense of joy in life. For these reasons, I feel that *The Oceanic Mind* continues the tradition of spiritual odyssey, but in a new key that eschews the authority and conviction typical of that genre and embraces the unreliability of the human narrator.

Somehow, in this unpretentious book, in which one can easily recognize oneself as an ordinary person growing up in a weird world, the tremulous voice of madness transcends its own implicit self-critique, suggesting to me a privileged opportunity for the interested reader, whether a mental health professional, a carrier of psychiatric diagnosis, or a curious bystander, to entertain an 'other', perhaps 'higher' level of emotional experience and existential truth.

Charles Levin, Ph.D
Supervising and training analyst
Canadian Institute of Psychoanalysis
Editor-in-chief
Canadian Journal of Psychoanalysis/Revue canadienne de psychanalyse

Preface

I HAVE LONG BEEN DIAGNOSED WITH BIPOLAR DISORDER.
I recognize and have experienced that bipolar disorder and schizo-phrenia are devastating illnesses. I have tried many alternate therapies after first having undergone conventional therapy and the medica-tions that were available in the early seventies. After a long search through alternate therapies, I continue with conventional medical care.

I have found that mental illness can be a doorway to other aspects of life. These aspects are recorded in various philosophies, but are generally unattainable by the average person. However, this does not detract from the fact that I have an illness that requires treatment.

There's an expression that to find salvation you need to search as someone whose hair is on fire looks for a pond of water. That's the type of motivation someone suffering from mental illness has.

As my illness proceeded, I found something beyond the turmoil that seemed oceanic or angelic, where there was a tangible connection between people and their spirits.

This is not a new concept. Carl Jung, who experienced a breakdown of sorts, coined the term *synchronicity.* It represents "meaningful coinci-dences." It speaks to a sense of order in the universe, an invisible hand that ties in with karma.

This book looks to provide new hope for people facing these con-ditions. Instead of having their sense of magical thinking dismissed, these people can be pioneers of new ways of viewing the world. Instead of thinking of themselves as human wreckages, they can under-stand that their conditions are not a result of lack of character and not a result of a shortage of willpower. Get help. Get on medication.

Medication has come a long way from the restrictive drugs of the not-too-distant past.

But also be aware that there is something majestic happening if you can separate the signal from the noise.

Childhood

Want to Land Up in the Douglas?

MY FATHER DECIDED TO NAME ME after both grandfathers. So I landed up with the same name as his father. In retrospect, I wondered if my father's relationship with his father reflected on me. I saw my father in church only for weddings. When I asked him about it, he said he got enough religion growing up. His father was a very religious man. From what little I know, and from reading about the area they lived in, he was considered eccentric. Today he would be considered a "born-again Christian." I have little information about how he grew up, but wonder how he felt about his father and whether having the same name had any effect on his reaction to me.

I recall a lot of arguments in the early years of my life. My father would intervene, often taking my side, but in a very heavy-handed way, alienating me from my siblings. My father would start the week with parental statements such as "Life is not a bowl of cherries." and "You shouldn't look at the world through rose coloured glasses." By Thursday, this would soften, and he was often out drinking with the boys and chasing women for the weekend. From a behavioural stand-point, growing up with this weekly cycle could be considered a basis for my own cyclic behaviour.

I was very hyper, with repeated phrases and insistent questions, and I would bug my father to the point where he would ask me in a loud voice if I wanted to land up in the Douglas. The Douglas was the last stop in psychiatric care on Montreal Island.

At one point I was left in the care of a baby sitter. She was about sixteen, I was about six. It was such a peaceful atmosphere. There was such a calmness that was very different than the usual family atmosphere. I loved my family very much but the dynamics were turbulent in contrast to what I experienced with this sitter.

When I was around seven years old, my mother would tell the pediatrician that I was much more active than my older siblings. He would say that I'm normal. But at one point she had me put on some medication. I only got worse and was soon taken off it.

Tennis Anyone?

I was visiting Toronto with my mother. We stayed with former neighbours, whose children were somewhat older than me. I was about ten years old, a bundle of energy, and quite a bit of a brat. I was still considered hyperactive, although this was never explained to me.

I was taken to play tennis with some of the daughter's friends. In the middle of it, I had a sense of coming alive and started to really enjoy myself. People responded in kind. I was treated like a king. My mood and sense of joy seemed to change the way I was treated in a very positive way. They let me steer the car on the way back. When I got out of the car, I remembered my life situation and couldn't keep up the state I was in. There was a sense that past behaviour needed to be consistent with the present. So I went back to being a brat, with regrets. But I never forgot the transformation.

Friday Nights at Home

I have a sister who is ten years older than me, a sister six years older, and a brother who is five years older.

I recall in my early teens that Friday night would be a very sad time for my mother. With my father absent, and me being the only one young enough to still be at home, I could feel my mother's sadness, like being immersed in a cold pool.

Early School Years

In gym class, if you did something wrong, inevitably that led to the gym teacher having you bend over and being hit with a tennis shoe, hard. I got hit in a tender place by a soccer ball and yelled out an obscenity. The gym teacher yelled out my name, and I said that I couldn't help it and that it just slipped out. He laughed. I didn't get the running shoe.

Years later I ran into the gym teacher in a bar, and he remembered that incident and was explaining that there was something wrong with me, with a friend of mine nodding his head in agreement. I didn't appreciate him bringing this up in front of an audience. I denied it, but later recognized some synchronicity in meeting up with him that one and only time, so long afterward.

In elementary school I could be given to spontaneous outbursts. I would make up words that I would repeat over and over, thinking it was quite cute. My social life took a beating. I was not a popular kid.

Making up phrases and repeating them has followed me all my life. I try to be discreet about it. When alone at home or driving a car, I can let loose with a torrent of phrases. There are times when it is irresistible, and during a different phase, I'm ashamed of it and have no desire to say them.

Ski Accident

When I was twelve, my parents went away to Washington together. This was a very unusual circumstance. It was winter, and my older siblings and I decided to go skiing. I ended the day racing down the hill, I hit a bump, and broke both bones in my left leg. I was hospitalized for a week. There was a Hong Kong flu scare then, and there were no visitors allowed.

At first I was upbeat. But as the week wore on, I couldn't keep my buoyant mood, and for the first time I fell into a deep depression. Even going to the drinking fountain became really difficult. I felt awkward and so unworthy. Other people seemed so together and adultlike. I had a sense of heavy judgment from inside and out.

The depression lasted a number of weeks. I had trouble falling asleep. All the manic words and behaviour from the past weighed heavily on me. I also found life took on a different tone. TV commercials seemed aimed at me and blended with my depressed mood. There was a sense of paranoia, a sense that there was a secret side of the world and human relations. In a commercial I would see an interaction between a child and his mother with sinister undertones of a power struggle and put-down. I had a sense of a loss of innocence, a sense that the world was fraught with danger and deception. Words and inflections took on multiple meanings. Words such as *high* or *low* in the middle of a sentence could take on a sense of pecking order and struggle to keep one another in their place, sort of a one-upmanship but at a more subliminal level, while people's awareness remained at a more mundane level.

Horse Camp

I was sent to a camp that did two things: taught you to ride a horse, tried to get you to become born-again. I went two summers in my early teens. The first summer I was rather manic and almost got kicked out. The second summer I was depressed. I took the horsemanship and the Bible very seriously.

When getting tested for horsemanship, I was put on a horse called Sico Sissy. We were to walk the horse one way toward an embankment, turn around and trot, then canter back.

Sico had had a long day. She walked faster and faster, and instead of turning around, she ran up the embankment, toward the barn. I had a flash of temper and turned her around in midflight, walked her down the embankment, trotted, and cantered back.

I passed the test. Many years later, I sometimes find my left hand gravitating a certain way. It's as if I am holding the reins of a horse. I call this "riding Sico Sissy." I remember it as a win, where I overcame the subconscious horse and got it to obey. I connected this hand movement only recently to the camp event. My interpretation has changed as a result. Rather than being concerned and distracted by unconscious movement, I interpret it as a positive indication that my body wants to "turn the horse around." I find it ironic that Sico Sissy was, at one time, a circus horse. If you kicked her in the right place she would kneel down or do other things. My horse was a trick pony.

This is part of the realignment of my thinking to some of my body language. Another example is when I focus on my breathing: often my throat closes momentarily. I originally interpreted this as an obstacle and resistance to monitoring my breathing. Now I see it as a sign that my muscles are nicely relaxed, and I gently continue to monitor my breath.

Catch You Later

I remember writing a note to a friend while in a fragile condition. At the end of it, I wrote *Catch you later*.... For some reason I really struggled with those words, even though it was a common phrase and one that we both used. It worried me.

When the friend got the note, he was really upset about the term *Catch you later*. I remember wondering if my focus on that phrase had any bearing on his response.

Psycho-Cybernetics

My parents got divorced. My mother went through a phase of looking for answers. She came back from one seminar with a book: *Psycho-Cybernetics* by Maxwell Maltz. He was a plastic surgeon who became fascinated with the overall changes to a person's life that could be the result of a nose job or some other cosmetic correction. Sometimes there was no change and the person acted as if they still had a deformity. He wrote about how the mind has a blueprint of a person's self-image. Self-help was useless unless the person believed it to be the truth about who they were.

My mother didn't mind me taking control of the book. I read it over and over. It made a lot of sense. One problem I had with it is that I was very different at different times, so I didn't know how to determine my self-image.

High School

I WAS A CLASSIC MANIC-DEPRESSIVE person in high school, in retrospect. I could go for long period of relative wellness, but I would eventually become hyper and childish. The depressions were eerie. I remember walking to band class and being in an area where no one was around. I relaxed for a minute, but the thought came up that I wasn't going to escape that easily. I had the sense of having parts of me that were silent but present.

I was seeing a psychiatrist during my early high school years. I had trouble articulating my situation to the doctor, but was able to convey my general anxiety while in a depressed state. I came out of my state of anxiety for a moment one day to ask for directions in the hospital where my mother worked. The person I asked for directions told my mother how confident and personable I was. When my mother told me this, I wondered about how it felt out of character but fit with my mother's wishes about me.

During a depressed state, I often confided in my brother-in-law. I remember one time he suggested I go skating, and I couldn't bring myself to do it. He couldn't understand the depths of my misery and how hard it was to be in public. It was difficult to get anyone to understand what it is like to be in a depression.

School was disastrous at these times. It seemed as though the whole world changed when I was depressed. I got the impression that teachers thought I was on street drugs. This was not the case. I don't even know if someone said anything to that effect or whether I just came up with it out of paranoia.

I played athletics. One time during a basketball practice, I burst into tears and left the building. I remember thinking on the way home that this was the worst life could get. Life couldn't get any worse. Little did I know what was in store for me.

When my mother found a psychiatrist for me to talk to, she wasn't very happy about it. There is a stigma that is very unwholesome about mental illness. Very few people knew about my condition or treatment. There is a myth about a person's character and worth and how this is tied to mental condition. My vindication is that drugs are now available that can help prevent the depths of illness involved.

The psychiatrist was a kindly person. The only subject that seemed to upset him was my mother. He mentioned a symbiosis between us. I think he had mother issues. My depression lifted on its own, and he proclaimed me cured. I wanted to continue seeing him, as I felt there was a much larger problem than we had talked about. Nope, the sessions were over. He pulled the plug.

College Years

I WENT INTO COLLEGE TAKING HEALTH SCIENCES. I took a hypnosis course that was offered. I secretly wanted to get hypnotized as a way of curing myself of the depression and the looming dark side energy that came with it. Each time I came down from a bout of manic phrases and childish behaviour, there seemed to be a very powerful anger lying just below the surface. At one point the teacher did a group hypnosis session on the class. I didn't get hypnotized, but kept my eyes shut and tried hard. The teacher knew his stuff and recognized that I was not in a trance, so finally I opened my eyes, feeling a bit sheepish.

I also took a "play the blues" course. College was fun back then, with elective courses outside standard curriculum. I aced this course, as I had been playing piano practically since birth. I had been playing the blues and playing in bands for years already.

Since I had few friends, the piano became a companion from an early age. I could get lost in the music and carried away emotionally. I recall being embarrassed about my emotions after playing without knowing why.

After flunking all my science courses and spending most of my time playing chess in the campus coffeehouse, I went to work at a local warehouse. I would head off in the morning as if I were going to school. That lasted a while, but my mother found out before the school year ended. She wasn't very happy about it, but recognized I appeared to have inherited the work ethic that both of my parents had.

I worked for a couple of years before going back to college. This time I applied the concepts of *Psycho-Cybernetics* and did very well. I am very persistent with methods and beliefs. In the span of years, I never forgot what I learned from that book, and when turning over a new leaf going to school, I put that knowledge into practise. I acted as if I were at the top of each class. The work became easy. My economics teacher looked at my text, saw my highlighting throughout, and recognized that I was working hard. But it was a labour of love. I was aiming for the top of the class, and I pulled it off in each class.

University Years

I DIDN'T DRINK DURING UNIVERSITY. I had quit the previous year, as I didn't drink very well. At varying levels of alcohol, I could black out and wake up the next day having no memory of the evening after a certain number of drinks. And it wasn't as if I went to sleep. I was generally a ball of grievous energy, acting out issues that I was barely aware of in a sober state. In the blacked-out state, huge concerns would surface that consciously were repressed.

I wondered about consciousness and who I really was. Who was there when I was blacked out? After many trials and tribulations, I quit drinking. Drinking was a theme that has cropped up in various forms in both sides of my family. My mother's father quit drinking. I don't know why he quit or what he was like before he quit. My father drank to excess against his family's wishes. In my experience, my father was very happy when drunk. I wanted to reach that state, but very seldom did. I don't miss drinking. It caused a lot of grief for me and my family.

First Year of University

I went to university in Ontario. I had spent one semester in Montreal and passed everything. However, my mother's husband got upset when I took ski socks off the basement clothesline for a ski day. I very seldom skied. In my house growing up, you wouldn't think twice about taking socks that were available. But it was a way for him to drive a wedge. It was an unlikely coincidence that the one day I went skiing, they were going too, and the socks were there for the taking. In later years I recognized it as a synchronistic event. It enabled him to tell me that "...as much as I love your mother, either you leave or I do." So I·chose a university in Ontario instead of in Montreal.

One of the first things I did at university was to join the skydiving club. I jumped seven times, but the last time I blacked out momentarily in midair when being tested for pulling my own rip cord. I landed wrong, spraining my knee and ankle. I was going to go back up, but thought about the blackout and decided against it.

During the first year, I lived at the house of an elderly lady quite a ways from the university. I didn't want to live in residence since I was a bit older, and also because I was, for the most part, using my own savings, and it was cheaper off campus.

I went home during Christmas. I gave the impression that things were going well, maybe too well. I had a sense that I couldn't keep it up. I hadn't made a lot of friends at school. I could feel the familiar sense of looming dark energy.

When I got back after Christmas, I started to feel turmoil in my emotions and thoughts indicating an impending bipolar crash. This time it was more potent than ever.

Instead of feeling depressed, my bipolar cycle had shifted. A fury welled up, and I felt it very physically. There was no physical acting out; this was internal. It reminded me of "brake loading" a car, where you press on the accelerator and the brakes at the same time.

I remember dodging this heavy black sensation from within and finally deciding to let it take over. I could feel the sticky heaviness in my brain and eyes. The poor lady I was living with was totally spooked when she saw me in this shape. So I fought it off once more. I don't know how to describe how I fought it off. It felt sort of like taking off a tight shirt. It involved attempting to think in my usual buoyant inner voice while keeping an inner eye out for the black energy. There was a sense of having an adversary. In later years I learned to think of it as a heavy assistant. This was reminiscent of a Buddha story about the evil counterpart showing up and being treated as a guest instead of trying to push him out.

I had no place in public. I was unacceptable. The thoughts and feelings were constant and on me like a wet blanket. Every step was accompanied by a flurry of brutal thinking.

The Yoga of Desperation

There was no let up. I kept going to school with very little ability to concentrate over the turmoil in my mind.

Through all of this, a strange thing happened. Through anguish, angels emerged. I started to see and get a reaction from a very sweet side of people. Years later I read about "the yoga of desperation," where, when under extreme duress, the mind has nowhere else to go, and it escapes into the upper echelon—the part yogis refer to when they greet each other with "Namaste."

There was a girl in one of my computer classes who was very receptive to me while in this upper echelon condition. At one point, the tumultuous energy part of me took over and approached this girl without saying a word.

She exclaimed, "Not you!"

What could she have meant by that?

At another time, I was sitting in a university dining area with very few people around. My mind was in its chronic state of turmoil. A girl sat down across from me and started talking and moving her hands. I found my mind calming down. She brought me back to my senses for a time, smiled, and left. I never saw her again.

I found a counselling service at the school and started getting regular, ineffective treatment. It did provide me with a sounding board, but I was clearly out of the therapist's league. I would talk about doublethink and how people seemed to communicate at various levels. She asked if I meant body language. Hardly.

In a computer course, we were given an assignment to write a hotel application. I had a computer message, "Guest Checks Out." My brutal mind latched on to this, and as the program listing scrolled down, and the phrase was encountered, I would have the physical sense of being a guest that was being checked out by the heavy energy inside. It took over in a very physical sense. I had a sense of being killed off by a part of me that was taking over and checking me out for good.

The counsellors were very excited about this and wanted to see the program, which, of course, was nothing special. It was an internal event.

The program ran fine as a simple hotel application. The message "Guest Checks Out" was a normal part of the running software program.

The counsellor gave me the name of a psychiatrist in Toronto to contact if and when I got there.

First Hospitalization

It became clear that there was going to be no letup of my illness during the second semester. I was advised to check into the hospital associated with the university.

This was my first hospitalization for the illness. I had no diagnosis or label to put on it. There was very little happening concerning the hospital treatment.

I recognized one girl on the ward who I had seen working in one of the libraries. I felt bad for her, as she was clearly in a fragile state. We were all drugged with the postwar cocktail of sedatives and anti-whatever medications that was available at that time. It felt like being on a planet with a heavy gravitation field. It didn't help the condition.

Just being out of the stress of everyday life was healing. I dropped two of my classes. I had previous credits from Quebec that would make up for these dropped courses within the three-year degree program. I started going to classes from the hospital. It went okay. I passed the remaining courses.

My oldest sister picked me up from the university. I was brought back to Quebec for the summer. My bed was installed in my sister's basement. My mother's second husband was convinced that I was only getting sick in order to come back to stay with my mother. He certainly had his own problems with bouts of anger that he used to turn on me. He eventually turned on my mother when there was no one else left. He wanted to make certain I didn't come back to stay at his home. I didn't really mind.

My mother was a nurse and approached a doctor on the psychiatric staff about my condition. I met with him once or twice. He was convinced that I would benefit from a new medicine, lithium. He explained that lithium was a mineral and was plentiful and cheap and very effective in dealing with manic depression, or what is now called bipolar disorder. It was the first time I had been given a diagnosis. He had me taking lithium tablets, as he felt they were more potent than capsules.

I wasn't sure that I was manic-depressive, since my world had become more of a schizophrenic journey during first-year university. I recognized that my early years were more of a classic manic-depressive phenomenon.

I worked two jobs that summer. I worked at the canning factory where my brother-in-law worked and as a packer for moving companies. I felt like my old self. I kept on the lithium. I stayed well.

Second- and Third-Year University

For the rest of my time at university, I stayed on the lithium and did not have any issues with the illness. In second year, I lived far from campus with someone into library science. I spent most of my time at school getting assignments done quickly and hanging out with a couple from Newfoundland. It was a fun time.

Occasionally, when under some duress, I could feel the dark energy start to emerge. I would then have a sense of damping it back down and having it go "back to sleep."

After second year, I moved closer to university, to a house that had students away for the summer. I was minutes from the campus. I moved into the nicest room, but was relegated to a tiny room in the basement when the soon-to-be doctors and physiotherapists returned.

During the break between second and third year, I worked for a moving company and continued to live off campus. I hired one of the Newfoundland friends and drove the truck. We had a third person from Russia who spoke very little English.

One time, I drove past a graveyard, honked the horn, and said, "Wake up the dead!"

The Russian understood this and found it very funny. But it wasn't manic. I didn't feel the urge to make up sounds and words.

I started seeing a girl who was also spending the summer in town. She became my girlfriend. This was my first long-term relationship.

I felt like I had left the illness behind. Very few people knew about it, and I didn't talk about it to family or friends. I just took my lithium and continued to do well.

There was on-campus recruiting happening in third year. I had decent marks and presented myself well. I was invited to second interviews with two departments of an oil company. I received offers from both.

One offer was for an internal area that was technical in nature. The other was with the chemical division, with an emphasis on how the business operated. I felt that the technology would always be changing, but the business requirements would remain more static. I joined the chemical division.

Oil Company

IT IS INTERESTING THAT THE BUSINESS I started my post-education career in was at the opposite end of the spectrum of what I cared about as a child. When I found out that Lake Saint-Louis in Montreal was polluted, I was very concerned about the lake and the planet. Going to Sarnia and seeing an open chemical pool in front of the oil company building was bothersome.

Do You Know What a "Golden Boy" Is?

I started off well. I was living with my girlfriend from university. We both got computer jobs in Toronto. Someone in the polymers group approached me about a data entry system that they were looking for. I was too naive to talk to my boss. I saw it as very similar to another existing application on the minicomputer that they were using. So I copied and adapted it and a week later presented it to the polymers guy. He was very impressed and let my boss's boss know. An analyst, who apparently had made some attempt at creating specifications, was not very happy. When I had my first performance review, my boss asked me if I had ever heard the term *Golden Boy*. I was succeeding.

Stopping Taking Lithium

I was feeling well and had been since first-year university. I heard from my mother that lots of patients feel that they don't need the medication any longer, once they feel well, and go off it and subsequently go off the edge of the known universe.

Much later I read that it was typical of the bipolar condition to have large gaps between episodes of sickness at the beginning. Episodes would happen more and more often, until a mixed-emotion state would become the norm with ongoing episodes of the disease.

I stopped taking lithium during the end of my first year at the oil company. There were no ill effects at first other than my hands were no longer shaky. My girlfriend and I had split up, and I had moved to an apartment alone.

I started seeing another girl from university who lived in Montreal. She would comment about how most people have a childlike side but mine seemed to be so much more pronounced. I had gone manic, along with a lexicon of silly phrases, and had a lack of awareness of the effect of my behaviour on the people around me.

I could feel the crash building. I got very worried and filled with dread. I had gone through such a fury in first-year university. I went to a walk-in clinic and got a prescription for lithium. It was too little, too late. The illness returned with a vengeance.

I got in touch with Dr. J, who was recommended by the university doctor. She put me on some medication and started the "talking cure."

I continued to work without a break. I continued to see my girlfriend. I would go to Montreal for a weekend every four weeks, and she would come to Toronto every other four weeks. So we would see each other every second weekend.

I would be a psychotic mess while at work and suddenly clear up at the train station when going to Montreal or picking up my girlfriend. I would be right as rain every second weekend. I would not question this transformation internally, as I didn't want to spoil the effect. It gave me hope that if the "unconscious horse" felt that good times were underway, the condition would evaporate. The condition wasn't something that just happened to me; there was control at some level.

This lasted about a year. My boss wondered what had happened to my productivity. I let him know I wasn't feeling well. So he had me come into his office, and we talked. He was clearly unimpressed with me. I was no longer considered a golden boy.

Second Hospitalization

AFTER ABOUT A YEAR, MY DOCTOR FIGURED OUT THAT I wasn't improving and was actually getting worse. The drugs were ineffective. Life was a nightmare. Visits with my girlfriend were no longer a holiday from my condition. She stayed with me through this rough period, but we split up not long afterward.

Double Sixes

I was advised not to return to work by Dr. J. There was no room in the hospital she was associated with, so I was on standby on the eighteenth floor of my apartment building with a view of Maple Leaf Gardens. I was in no condition to read or follow the TV, so I brought out the backgammon board and sat at my kitchen table and played myself.

I had the sense of my ideal self playing against my troubled self. As always in this condition, the curtain between the conscious self and the subconscious seemed to have been lifted. I got a sense of correlation between thinking and the roll of the dice.

I was using a backgammon cup to hold the dice. At one point, I had a sense of certainty and said aloud, "Double sixes."

I rattled the cup and rolled double sixes. I performed this three times in a row and then put down the cup with a sense of calm. I didn't have the feeling that I could call on this at any time, like ordering coffee. I wasn't sure what the lesson was. Of course, it could have been coincidence, but that's what happened. And to me it was a meaningful coincidence. I spent some time after this, when playing backgammon, trying to control the dice, but the results were underwhelming. These days I don't consider it a worthwhile pursuit. I think the lesson was learned. The world is magical but capricious. We're here to work on ourselves collectively and individually.

During this time I was very impressed with my ideal self. It seemed to have come alive and was all that I wanted to be. I was once again reminded of *Psycho-Cybernetics* and how you can recognize the truth that you are free to be, focus on, and evolve as your ideal self. In the book, it also advised that for about twenty-one days there would be the sense of dual energy systems as the mind/body gets used to the new self-image and lifestyle. I found this insightful in that I experienced dual energy systems, and it was not only a function of mental illness.

Nobody is That Good

When I talked to Dr. J about my ideal self, she was dismissive. "Nobody is that good." she said. I don't know what motivated her to respond that way.

As was always the case, when it came time to be admitted to the hospital, a huge anger welled up.

The first night was a tumultuous affair. I was in an internal rage. I never acted it out; it was only an internal fit. The nurses noticed the bottled-up rage, and Dr. J assured them that I wasn't violent.

Once again the hospital environment provided a stress-free shelter. I eventually regained my health and enjoyed the hospital experience with the staff and patients.

Back to Work

It was difficult going back to work.

My second performance review was very different. I refused to sign until they took out a sentence, something about that we are all responsible for our own health. As was explained to me sometime later, it wasn't as if I had a sore foot.

I stayed on my medication, which at this point didn't include lithium. I no longer had a girlfriend. I had few friends. And it wasn't long before I was once again immersed in a chronic psychotic episode. I don't even recall going manic beforehand.

Third Hospitalization

I HUNG ON AS LONG AS I COULD. I started hanging out with a cousin who was a doctor. He eventually gave me a strong dose of chlorpromazine, which my doctor had me on. When I woke up the next morning, I still felt the physical effects of the drug and could barely sit up. I called my doctor and was admitted.

This time Dr. J had the idea that what was needed was a long-term stay in the hospital. There was a group of us who were there for months and got along very well. It was like being in a summer camp. None of us seemed terribly unwell during this time. The pressure was off.

I surmised that my condition was aggravated by my performance at work. If I maintained my equilibrium and didn't go manic and performed well at work, I might be okay. I thought back on the effect of lithium. It was useless once I was in a psychotic episode, but it seemed to be effective in preventing me from going manic. The manic behaviour enraged the part of me that was dominant during any subsequent episode.

I asked Dr. J to put me on lithium, and she listened to me. I stayed on it for years.

Your Job Has Been Moved to Calgary

I was on long-term disability in the hospital. When I got out, I wasn't welcomed back to work. I received a letter stating that my job had moved to Calgary, even though the chemical division that I was in had stayed in Toronto. I declined to move, as expected.

Live for Today

I kept in touch with people I met in the hospital. There was one girl I was seeing. There was another girl whom I found very attractive. I drifted away from the first girl and started seeing Jill, who was nine years older than me.

The first girl went into a depression and jumped in front of a subway. Someone contacted Jill, who informed me. My involvement felt like a weight around my neck. The normal rules didn't seem to apply. If you stop seeing someone, the results can be lethal.

There was another guy I was friends with in the hospital who also committed suicide around this time. One of his acquaintances found my number in his address book and called to inform me. I hadn't gotten together with him for a long time. Somehow the sad news always seemed to make its way back to me.

I was living with a friend from Montreal, but spent most of my time at Jill's apartment. Although I didn't drink in university, after multiple hospitalizations, I had started up again. It was more out of futility than anything else since my life was in the Dumpster most of the time. It had become a "live for today" experience.

Jill and I would put on music tapes, have some beer, and have a lot of fun.

She was classic bipolar, and we both went manic together. She loved the words I came up with. Jill had two cats that I renamed Teco and Crabby Guts. She had an apartment-size piano with the music for "Poor Butterfly" on it. Upon reflection, I consider "Poor Butterfly" to be a whimsical description of Jill overall. We listened to a lot of Abba and André Gagnon.

We would get drunk and a bit reckless. I once called up the White House at 2 am to speak to the President. I did get through to someone from security, and I'm sure the phone number is on a list somewhere down south. I called up a guy who I was friends with in university. I liked the guy. For some reason I called at 3 am and taunted him on the phone. I bugged him about not having a girlfriend. This was ironic since I spent most of my teens without one. I haven't talked to him since. I doubt I'll ever go to a reunion. I feel very bad about it thirty years later.

I landed a position with a placement agency. This was a salaried position that didn't pay well and had no security, but this was the arrangement, and I was given a position as a software developer in a real estate company.

The real estate company paid for the amount of processing time they used. I had a boss who was very hard to get along with. I worked on a system that was well written, but unfinished. The person leaving probably couldn't stand the boss. All I had to do was come up with a third stream of income for this treasury flow-of-funds program. One day the boss gave me a torn corner of a page with a number on it. He said I had better be able to balance to that amount in production or else. It didn't balance. I spent that evening putting in traces and running the program over and over. It wouldn't balance.

The next morning, the first thing the boss did was to have a minion check on my computer usage. He screamed at me that if I ran the program one more time, I was fired. I told him that it didn't balance. I asked if it might be because the number was wrong.

He said, "So you think we have a problem with the general ledger? Well I better see about that!" So he called and asked what the balance was for the day before. I watched his ears turn pink, and he said over the phone, "You owe an apology to a programmer here!"

He had the value for the wrong date. My results were bang on. He's the one who should have apologized.

The whole scene upset my fragile state. I never returned to that job. Instead I slipped into a walking psychosis. But I got the job done. I ran into someone from that project a year later who said the flow-of-funds program ran without a hitch.

Walk In the Woods

I went for months trying to cope with the latest episode. My thoughts were jagged and hysterical. At one point Jill and I went for a walk. We walked towards a park beside a wooded area. I somehow reasoned with my mind and got it to settle down. My condition cleared up magnificently. I was right in the moment. Jill and I walked on a path into the wooded area. I marvelled at the green grass and trees. It lasted about a half hour. As we left the woods I tried to hold onto the state of mind. This caused the turbulence to start back up again and I was soon deep in the midst of my chattering mind. But I never forgot that walk in the woods.

Jill found a job as a receptionist in a construction site north of Toronto. I was visiting her there when the chatter in my mind reached a crescendo and I panicked. I felt my mind turn on me. I drove my car back into town and parked it across from the hospital and broke down in tears as I went through the process of re-admittance.

Fourth Hospitalization

ONCE AGAIN THE HOSPITAL ENVIRONMENT lifted me back up. I was first diagnosed as a borderline personality. This was later changed to bipolar II. Much later my condition was diagnosed to be bipolar with schizoaffective disorder. I think that in my late teens, my subconscious left the depressive part of the manic-depressive cycle for the uncharted waters of psychosis, with a self-directed fury that reached a peak when admitted to the hospital.

My condition was accompanied by awareness. I was in the eye of the storm, with a part of me keeping sane, allowing me to go to work and perform between thought interruptions and energy bursts.

I had the sense of one or more parts of my personality attempting to drive the proverbial bus, sometimes two at a time wrestling for the steering wheel. It reminded me of a Walt Whitman poem where he proclaims that he contains multitudes. It also reminded me of a Bible passage where a guy named Legion had multiple demons that were cast into pigs so he could regain his senses.

I prefer Walt's version.

For some reason, when I was not in the hospital, it was very difficult to meet and establish a girlfriend. In the hospital it was very easy. This time, I fell for a young lady named Gail.

The hospital had varying stages, from stage one, constant observation, through to stage four, coming and going from the hospital pretty much independently.

While on stage four, I went to visit Jill and told her I didn't think we were healthy together. I broke up with her. We walked around the block after I announced this decision. She kept wanting to hold hands, and I felt very bad about the decision, but considering the state we both had landed up in, I considered it the right choice and stuck to it.

Fatherhood

Gail and I got into a relationship. We had a child together, a boy we named Eric. I offered to live with her or get married.

She said, "It's the eighties. Single mothers are normal. You can bring gifts on his birthday or something."

The baby was born at the same hospital. By then I was out and on a contract back at the real estate company, doing something completely different within the information technology spectrum. I got the news of his birth by phone. Gail had gone for a stress test, and they found the baby struggling and immediately induced labour. He was three months premature, weighing two pounds and seven ounces. He was in an incubator, or as we called it, "a womb with a view." Eric lived in the incubator for three months. Gail was there every day rubbing his back.

Gail lived on the far west side of the town, I was still living with my friend from Montreal on the east side. I was driving an old MGB sports car back and forth across town. When I was growing up, I had a neighbour who always had an MGA or B in his driveway and tinkered with it. It was like fulfilling a dream buying one. It turned out to be dependable transportation, but I didn't put any money into it, and I was eventually pulled off the road by a cop in the pouring rain with one windshield wiper broken. I had to have it towed away and never saw it again.

Jill became a patient at the hospital during that time. She had fallen into a deep depression. While waiting to visit the baby, I went up and sat at a table in the familiar psych ward. Jill saw me, and the colour drained from her face. We didn't speak. That was the last time I saw her. She jumped off her mother's balcony. I found out from Dr. J, who asked if I wanted to talk about it. I couldn't. It was a sad day when I phoned her mother to offer my condolences. Jill deserved better. I still think of her, like a flower in a meadow beautifully in bloom.

Coping Techniques

The placement agency didn't want me to continue contracting through them when I returned from the hospital. The lady I was dealing with was nice enough to introduce me to Mike, to find a full-time position. When I asked why him, she said, "Because he's the best."

He was British and took me to a local British pub for bangers and mash. He was aware of my condition and offered an ability that he considered useful: when you are having a heated discussion with someone, picture yourself watching in a high corner of the room.

I had already developed a number of coping techniques. I had learned to breathe into my diaphragm in long breaths. I would focus on sounds and the sights around me. I would play piano for hours, which was a fantastic catharsis. But as long as there was the sense that I wasn't performing well at work and needed to work to survive, there was pressure. Somehow work and the world of men became important when part of me was furious with myself.

It Appears to be a Lung

My father retired in the late seventies. He had a trailer to travel in and spend the summer in Montreal, and a bigger trailer in Mesa, Arizona, where he spent the winter.

We both were musical. He played the accordion by ear, and I played the piano by my ear.

As a child, at one point, I developed an interest in automobiles. I pointed out the solenoid to a neighbour, who was impressed and told my parents that I seemed to have a talent for mechanics. My father was scornful. He wanted me to go to university, not become a mechanic.

My father used to cut my hair. He continued to overcome my wails of protest and cut my hair to the bone. He would remark to us that it would be great to be a barber and be your own boss. I tried many times to follow this advice on various business ventures. My wife and I are still trying.

My father phoned me not long after my son was born, to tell me that he had been diagnosed with lung cancer.

Coincidentally, I got a contract with Ontario Cancer Research. It was a short contract tracking the demographics of cancer in Ontario. There were no big breakthroughs happening. I remembered the Crosby, Stills, and Nash song: "It appears to be a long...time." Instead the lyrics for me were: "It appears to be a lung," with an image of a group of surgeons standing over an open chest, looking in. They seemed helpless to do anything to remedy the situation. This was a version of the song I had come up with years before, as part of my manic repertoire of words and music.

My father returned to Toronto and lived in his own apartment

The only time I saw my father play the accordion was when he had a beer in front of him. His repertoire was from the coal-mining community in the Rockies where he grew up. When I was young he used to tell me that I was going to play accordion for him when he was old and blind. He never went blind, but he was in the final stages of lung cancer. He no longer could drink. I took out the accordion, to his protest, and played one of his songs, "Saturday Night Waltz." He challenged me to play "Clarinet Polka." I picked my way through it.

He said, "Why don't you get the sheet music? Give me that thing," and played the song. That was the first time I saw him play sober and the last time I saw him play.

I have that accordion today. I can still play "Saturday Night Waltz." My wife likes me to take it out and play it at parties. I play some Edith Piaf for her. My son-in-law, who I have been helping out on piano, also has tried playing it. The accordion case still has a list of songs written down in my father's handwriting. It's a great party instrument, as my father well knew.

While my father was admitted to the hospital for the last time, I was having an episode, despite having continued to take lithium. I read an article in *Reader's Digest* about a treatment for cancer. I got in touch with my father's doctor and talked him into contacting a research centre in Atlanta, although there was no hope. My father phoned me and told me to leave his doctor alone. He added that the doctor mentioned that I seemed very bright. This fit into my father's image of me.

OnQ

WHILE PLAYING CHESS WITH THE LOCAL BARBER, a fellow came in and we started talking. Pete was involved with a software developer in creating an interface between IBM PCs and telex machines. I was on the second contract at the real estate company and got involved in my spare time. Pete had his own home a block away from where I lived. So I got possession of this clunky portable IBM PC. I got it just after my room was burglarized, with the only thing stolen being a Commodore 64 computer. Good exchange.

I came up with the name OnQ (pronounced "On Q"). I usually come up with the names of my pets and companies.

While John, the other partner, wrote the communications layer to work with a British company's telex hardware, I wrote a word processor. The computer language, Turbo Pascal, was state-of-the-art at the time, and I found some freeware that was a complete word processor. I was very impressed with the code and wondered if I was in the right profession with wizards around creating freeware such as this. I did do something that no one appeared to have duplicated at the time, however. To fit with the thirty-eight or so character width of telex output, I provided the ability to mark a document, such as a spreadsheet, so that it could be output in slices. That was my main contribution.

We acquired a free office space in a building that was soon to be demolished. My contract ended, and I was getting paid by John and got a home improvement loan to keep going.

The stress of my father's condition and the stress of starting a new business got to me. I quickly fell into my thoughts and energy levels. The energy levels were reminiscent of Walt Whitman's phrase "I sing the body electric." Fantastic amounts of energy would course up my spine, through my chest, arms, and head. In later years I found this to be a gift as well as a curse. I tend to keep my hand and feet clenched when this energy is coursing, but when I become aware of it and let go, it is grounding.

My father died a stoic death. He and I joked to the nurses that when they were draining fluids from his lungs, it was all the beer that had gone down the wrong way throughout the years.

He passed away at seventy-three years old. My siblings were brought together and, at our invitation, my mother joined us, as we were all having trouble coping.

For the first time since before university, I was able to come out of my episode without having to be hospitalized.

There is a sense of justice in the dark energy I have described. Going through the authentic mourning of my father's condition and death seemed to have appeased this part of me. I recall an earlier example, when I was in high school, where I was in a similar but much lighter condition. I was trying out for the basketball team and did a decent job of playing defense. The heavy feeling lifted as a direct result. This part of me wants me to be a man and do a decent job of it.

Property Management Company

ONQ NEVER MADE ANY MONEY. Pete and I took a trip to England and met with the hardware people. They liked the slicing of spreadsheets, and the product did what we said it would do. They had something similar in their catalogue for Macs, and I saw it as a good alternative for IBM PCs. For some reason, we were good at getting the software ready, but not very good at marketing it and landing a deal.

The money to live on from OnQ was running out. I called a placement agency that I had contracted out of. They had a customer who was looking for a full-time project leader. Their business was residential and commercial construction and property management across North America. I got the job.

I continued to stay on lithium and nothing else. I seldom visited the psychiatrist except to get my prescription filled. I felt fine.

I had a good boss and hired a team to build residential and commercial software. I had found at OnQ that I enjoyed directing programming efforts, and I was promoted to property management development manager after a couple of years.

During this time, I had only one brush with a bipolar episode. I won a contest to go down south. I took an accountant lady with me since I was single at the time and she was interested. Her mood got ugly when we got there, for some reason. I found myself in the grips of a bipolar episode. I was like that for the whole week. It cleared up as I boarded the plane back home. I was fine after that.

The company hit hard times in the early nineties. I had built up a good team and was asked to come up with an ordered list of who to lay off. Being new to this, I said they were all really good and I couldn't think of anyone to lay off. None of them were laid off. I was laid off.

As luck would have it, a true head-hunter called around the company about a week before I was laid off. She recruited me for a software house in Markham, north of Toronto. I got the job about two weeks after being laid off.

Home Sweet Home

WHEN I FIRST MET GAIL, SHE CONSIDERED ALCOHOL to be voluntary retardation. During our long stay in the hospital, she was doing really well. When Eric was finally out of the hospital, he lived with her.

My friend from Montreal researched the market and bought a house. He didn't consult me. When I moved to the house my friend bought, he became my landlord and things got tense. We were not getting along.

There was one long driveway where I had my MGB parked in front of his Ford Zephyr. He also had a Mustang in Montreal. He told me if I needed to get my car out, he kept spare keys in his sock drawer. He went to Montreal to get his Mustang.

I went to get my car to go to Gail's on the other side of town. I looked all through the sock drawer and couldn't find the keys. I was very unhappy about it and decided to take the streetcar across town. It took nearly an hour. When I got to Gail's, there was a phone call waiting for me. It was the provincial police saying that my friend had run out of gas near Oshawa and wanted me to get my car and pick him up. It was difficult to explain to the dispatcher that I couldn't find the keys and wasn't about to take a streetcar back to the east side and resume my search of his sock drawer.

He made it home without my help. He was furious. When I got home, he had taken my graduation photo that I had in the living room and threw it on my bed. So I could see that there was no question of whose house it was.

I cashed in some bonds from the oil company days. The interest rate had been 19 percent when I bought them. I had enough for a high-ratio down payment on a semidetached house in the east end. I bought at a good time. Gail and Eric moved in.

In retrospect, the tension between my friend and I manifested in a way that fit his view that I wasn't a loyal friend and my view that his demands were unreasonable.

It was also a means for me to get up the motivation to buy my own house. That home tided me over in some very rough times. I was able to survive times I was in a state where I couldn't work and times where attempts to start a business had failed and the bills needed to be paid. I kept the house for over twenty years.

Separation

Gail and Eric moved into my house but we didn't do too well living together. She moved out with Eric in the late eighties. She lived on mother's allowance plus an agreed monthly payment from me that went to the government. In other words, she received the same amount whether I paid support or not.

I always made my payments. I would see Eric on weekends or evenings. There was no court order as to who had custody. We were on good terms, helping each other out and both involved with raising Eric as best we could.

Despite her previous view of alcohol, Gail took up drinking in a big way.

Her father was an alcoholic. She was prone to depression. So I guess that made her unipolar. She sometimes talked about committing suicide. She said I got her laughing and that helped.

We shared the same family doctor, who was Eric's doctor since birth. Dr. Y was very down-to-earth and compassionate. She would not put Gail on certain medications because Gail had a tendency to abuse medication.

From the late eighties through to the early nineties, I was doing okay. Gail had plenty of friends, drinking buddies mostly. She was very good at making friends. We remained friends as well, helping each other out as best we could.

Software House and Beyond

I CONTINUED TO TAKE LITHIUM. I was in an entirely different style of business in the software house in Markham. There was an office in Dallas that threw political grenades whenever the opportunity arose. It was the early nineties, and although I wasn't going over the edge, I was not in great shape. I much preferred my earlier job with the property management company.

For a vacation, I took Eric to a summer resort in the Muskokas that had a series of log cabins. Eric had developed tics. One was to scrunch his neck down and up again. By coincidence, a child psychiatrist was in the next cabin. His advice was to be very gentle when asking Eric about the tics. It was good advice, as I was very impatient with Eric when he was doing this.

It was a nice vacation. There was a three-legged race where Eric just jumped onto one of my feet and hung on to my leg while I ran to the finish line.

Back on the Street

I STARTED TALKING TO A FRIEND of a friend, Tony. He claimed to be in marketing and was looking to start a business. Since I was miserable where I was, I quit my job and joined him on the street.

I was very naive about what software I could develop in what time frame. Tony was concerned about a sales system. I gave it the name Sales Force One, which Tony liked. I was more concerned about building something that could be used to track time and activities. I was also interested in interfacing to a computer-assisted software engineering tool (CASE) so that you could model what you are building and press a button and a graphical software program was instantly available.

I got the CASE interface working well enough to demonstrate it. But the scope of what I built was all over the map, and the sales system was not to be found. I struggled for months on the software. I became manic trying to piece it together. Finally Tony came one day and severed the relationship. He was through with the partnership. I came down with a crash.

My energy tied me up, and the thoughts raced. I went for a long walk. I had a golden retriever named Fortune who got to go on lots of walks, as I found exercise to be of value in this condition. She was a very lucky dog and a good companion. Her good looks offset the look of grim determination that was on my face as I walked for hours around the neighbourhood.

It was August, and there were a lot of mountain ash trees in bloom. The orange berries seemed significant to me. Orange was, since early childhood, a favourite colour. I walked and observed the speeding and clashing thoughts. I marvelled at the colour orange. I was a wreck. It was a continuation and extension of what I went through in the early and mid-eighties.

I got in touch with Dr. J, who was reaching the end of her career. She had the same office, but it was full of frogs. This is what she was collecting. More on that later.

Chiropractic

MY SON WAS GOING TO KARATE lessons on the Danforth. Just down the street was a bookstore with an advertisement in the window about a psychic. So I went in and, on a whim, got a reading. This was prior to Tony ending the partnership, and my subsequent crash. According to her, I was going to make a lot of money and that I cared too much what people think.

My mind was very murky and had been since the software house job. I started going to this psychic as a sort of therapy. The therapy wasn't going to happen, but she did tip me off about a new type of chiropractic that, in her opinion, was very effective in a holistic way.

So I started to see the chiropractor she had told me about. It involved light touch at the base of the spine and the neck. There was a sea of tables, and people were encouraged to moan and writhe and breathe in a certain way while the chiropractor performed his touch. He was an expert at detecting and promoting energy states. I never entered the same state twice, but four or five times, I experienced life-changing states. And the chiropractor would be right there to witness and let me know I was in "stage nine" or whatever.

I spent years and tens of thousands of dollars following this approach, and I don't regret it, as it took me to places that very few people are aware of.

Since I tended to talk about my mental condition, the chiropractor recommended someone who had talking groups. There was a men's group one night a week and a mixed group another night.

Men's and Mixed Groups

THESE GROUPS WERE STARTED by a medical doctor who believed in Buddhism and therefore reincarnation. As part of his approach, he taught me how to breathe into my diaphragm. He had started a men's group and mixed group that was led by a colleague.

The groups were somewhat effective in socializing and energy work. There was one particular leader that had a Welsh background. I found him to be very perceptive about energy states and synchronicity.

The original doctor was adamant about getting me off medication. He more or less said that one needs to remove the surly bonds of medication in order to achieve higher energy states and live a fulfilled life. The original doctor remarked after one session that he could see in my energy field that the medication was keeping me from reaching the goal of self-realization. I stayed on my lithium just the same.

Men's Group Discussion

One evening I had a conversation with one of the guys in the men's group. I mentioned that I was Welsh and Irish, and possibly a little bit Scottish, but I didn't know much about that. The person I was talking to started expounding the virtues of being Scottish. He maintained that I should be very proud of any Scottish background. He mentioned that the thistle is the flower of Scotland. This seemed very meaningful to him, and I made a mental note of this.

Driving on the Highway

I was driving a red Toyota SR5. In my head was a whirlwind of thought, a lot of it abusive toward myself. It was a rant that started back up again as soon as I woke up each morning while in this phase. Somehow, driving never presented a problem for me, regardless of my internal state.

I noticed a black Toyota SR5 of the same year as mine on the road. It had a bumper sticker that proclaimed the owner was Scottish and to "Kiss My Thistle." It was a bold statement, and I took in the colour of the car, the attitude and considered it a valuable lesson. I had been told that I care too much what people think, and in my polarities, I was uncomfortable with the colour black.

This car indicated the opposite attitude, that I should be proud of my heritage and who I am.

There It Is Again

While visiting at my nephew's condominium years later, I noticed a black Toyota SR5 with a faded but legible bumper sticker. It was the same car. It was parked in the handicapped spot. I thought that was ironic. I felt that it was a continuation of the statement to be proud of my heritage, to keep a spunky attitude even though I had a handicap that had decimated my life and career.

Group Activities

So we would sit around on pillows in this room in Parkdale and talk and try to cry. There was a plastic bat to be used to get angry and hit a pillow with. I mostly saw inauthentic displays of anger.

One time, one of the guys in the mixed group really did get angry. He was ostracized by the group. He had previously told a story about a different group he was in where he had a disagreement with the others and was asked to leave the group. He took it very hard. So his self-image seemed to have been reinforced by this scenario. I found the group's reaction to be extremely hypocritical and I quit not long afterward.

Back to the Chiropractor

THE CHIROPRACTIC SESSIONS didn't help my condition. In fact, I felt less grounded. The chiropractor didn't seem to understand how I could get into a higher energy state and experience the unconditional love and still be stuck in a lower energy state afterward.

At one point I was deeply troubled, with my mind so bound up that even the rough side of my personality was looking for a way out. I lay down on the adjustment table and was told to breathe in short, rapid breaths. I found myself going into a state of total relaxed energy.

I felt as though I was hovering above my body. There was very little thinking. Any thought that passed through felt like a perturbation of the energy field. This lasted a few minutes, but the physical aftereffect lasted longer. When I opened my eyes, they appeared to focus much more clearly. People looked angelic. It felt oceanic. It was similar to the state I fell into in university, but more peaceful and with less awareness of my body and more awareness of the energy state. I felt peace of mind, but I also felt some struggle to go back to the familiar state of the union.

I took a walk and went to a local restaurant. Along with the calmness, I felt a little uneasy.

I went back to the chiropractor's office an hour later, feeling somewhat distant. The chiropractor asked if I was okay, and I replied that I was. I felt the thoughts creeping back in and my body tensing up. It was not long before I was back to the old condition.

After that time, I longed to return to that oceanic state of being on an energy plane. But most of the subsequent visits were stubbornly useless. My life continued to be plagued by multiple lines of thought and difficulty focusing on anything else. I could get a sort of a break if I did nothing. If I lay on my bed and just listened to the thinking, it could settle down. But when I reached for the doorknob, I would have the sense of two parts of my mind/energy reaching for it.

The only kind of reading I was able to concentrate on was self-help or philosophy books. In *The Path to Love* by Deepak Chopra, I found a very interesting summary about karma. He wrote on pages 194–195:

> The proof of karma doesn't lie in reward and punishments handed out by a cosmic judge. When people casually refer to "good karma" or "bad karma," they are confusing karma with reward and punishment, but the working of karma is much more profound...Our karma throws us into the roles of saint and sinner, man and woman, king and peasant, but these roles are temporary and shifting. None of them is really us. Spirit uses these roles the way a dramatist uses actors...Why do we play these roles? For experience, for growth, to find our way back to God. Ultimately, all karma serves only two purposes: either it is a sign of love from spirit or it is a lesson meant in love.

He wrote about reaching a stage where your wishes would manifest automatically. This reminded me of Joseph Campbell writing about how he went to visit a guru and how things got easier as he proceeded. Doors were opening to bring him in contact with this person. In other words, synchronicity was more apparent when getting closer to self-actualization.

The Zoo

WHILE UNDER CHRONIC DURESS, I decided to take Eric to the zoo. My friend from Montreal came along. I fought to keep my thinking straight, and we went ahead. I had a breakthrough where, in the midst of turmoil, I emerged into a peaceful oceanic atmosphere where everyone seemed angelic. But I was not on firm ground.

I felt magical. I tried to put a quarter in a drinking fountain and get Eric to find it. Eric would have nothing to do with it. Instinctively, he knew it was contrived.

We got on the mini-train, and I felt like the world was coming apart. I felt as though I was having a strong effect on the people around me, and I panicked. I left with Eric, with my friend following. We didn't even leave by the gate, we just walked straight to where the car was. I didn't know where the car was, I just walked there. My friend drove back to the east end of Toronto, where Eric and his mother lived at the time. I was slapping my hand on the side of the car, trying to break the spell, and endured what felt like the universe collapsing around me.

I dispatched my friend and Eric to go to the restaurant/tavern where Gail usually was, and I went in the opposite direction, crossed a few streets, and found Gail in the middle of nowhere with her boyfriend. He was a big guy, but I told him to leave, and he did. I took Gail for a coffee and explained my plight. She suggested that I had gotten too sick to carry on, and she accompanied me to the hospital.

Hospital Revisited

THIS WAS MY LAST TRIP TO THE SAME HOSPITAL. It was no longer a summer camp atmosphere. I think government cuts were having an effect on morale, and the nurses seemed agitated.

I was lining up for medication the first evening when a voice in my mind said that the nurse was going to say, *"You're good."* I felt nervous about the voice in my mind. It seemed very sure of itself.

The nurse issued the medication in silence. When it came to my turn, I took the medication, and she said, "You're good." This terrified me.

I went to my room, threw myself at the chest of drawers headfirst, and blacked out. I woke up strapped to the bed for the first time. I was out of the episode. I was not very happy. But I no longer felt the dual thinking.

Change of Plans

GAIL MOVED ONCE AGAIN. This time she moved into the basement of a house. You entered into the kitchen. The living room, bedroom and bathroom were behind that with only one door at the front. It was a firetrap. Gail had gotten to the point where all she seemed concerned about was drinking and her drinking buddies.

I contacted a lawyer to try to get custody of Eric. He told me that it would cost me a lot of money and I would not win.

I continued to see Eric as much as I could. I was going in and out of episodes.

Eric had friends who were playing hockey at the local arena. I signed him up, and away he went. He was small in stature, but not in heart. He was a fan of the Maple Leafs hockey team goalie Felix Potvin. In fact, he named one of his cats Potvin.

So he tried out at playing goaltender. I was generally not okay and remember one particular situation early on in the hockey practices. Eric was in nets. I was a mess. They were miles ahead of the competition and ran up the score to over 20–2 or so. I was convinced that my own runaway wishes were causing an imbalance in the score. I left the arena, went to my car in the parking lot, and prayed that the spell would be broken. I felt as if life as I knew it was over and my thoughts were potent and out of control. That was the kind of state I was in. This is what a psychiatrist would refer to as *magical thinking.*

I have no argument that I had succumbed to magical thinking in this case. I recognized my condition soon afterward, when I was told Eric's team played together in street hockey as well as on ice and were genuinely better, no help from me. It was a relief to realize this.

Gail eventually could not pay her rent and lost her place. All of her and Eric's worldly possessions were put in the backyard for nature to take its course. She finally let me take Eric. She had a number of cats. It started with a single cat, but she couldn't get it together to get them fixed, and there were more than ten cats roaming around when she lost the place. I took them in, and Eric and I had a terrible time with the idea that some or all of the cats couldn't stay. We finally settled on three cats staying, and I gave away the rest.

Breaking the Ice

I WAS INTRODUCED BY GAIL to a nurse who had a dog. We agreed to take our dogs for a walk along Ashbridges Bay by Lake Ontario. I was in a sensitive state and reading a lot of double meanings into conversations. A phrase she used was "to break the ice." It was a way of saying something to get to know each other. When we went on the walk, she again said, "… to break the ice." This seemed meaningful to me.

So we went on the outside of the peninsula, where the water was crashing into the rocks. We skipped stones, and the dogs ran free. We walked in the park to the bay part, which was covered with ice. Sure enough, my dog went through the ice and was swimming around, not sure what to do next. Well, I wasn't about to watch my dog drown. So I walked deliberately up to the dog, took her collar, and pulled her back onto the ice, and we walked back.

A week later there was a front-page story in the *Sun* magazine about some guy falling into the icy water and drowning trying to save his dog.

Mike Lands Me a Job

I HAD FAILED AT MY ATTEMPT at having a partnership with Tony. I was out of work with no means of support.

Mike, from the placement agency, called. He was living in England, but was in town to do some headhunting and put together some cash. He was living for free at a colleague's house, but I thought that he would be a good influence on Eric and I, so he moved into the basement.

I think Eric and I both benefitted from having Mike around. Mike would create little projects for Eric, like pairing socks after a wash. He introduced Eric to Dilbert cartoon books.

I helped Mike a bit, as he was feeling down about providing for his family so far away. I asked him who could love his children as much as he did, and he replied that no one could. That helped his resolve and also made me feel that I could be of value as a friend.

Mike had a database of candidates on a Macintosh that he was selling. I programmed an equivalent in Windows, but it was the information that was being sold rather than the platform it ran on.

Mike got me a job. The placement agent told me how Mike had effectively settled a dispute with a large client of theirs. He had a lot of respect for Mike's opinion. The respect might have taken a beating, as I was in a state of disrepair from the onset.

I was working with a bright fellow who started out as a nuclear physicist, but like a lot of people, found more lucrative work in information technology. I had trouble understanding the system. My ability to concentrate was greatly impaired.

I would lean on the physicist to get my job done. He became somewhat of a friend. We got together a few times at my place or his. He was a very bright fellow with a lot of integrity.

My condition got worse. I started to get a familiar sense that conversations around me had double meanings. I could feel the body electric out of control.

One time in the cafeteria, I decided to direct my energy to someone about ten or twelve feet away.

He bent over and softly said, "You're not going to get me."

I was very impressed with his response. I think he was from India or Pakistan. I passed him in the stairwell afterward, and he said I was going through a phase. I didn't say a word. I got the sense that he told me not to worry and I was on the right path.

Another very strange situation was when I couldn't sit at my desk and I went down to the cafeteria and sat down. Three people sat down at the next table. For about four sentences, I got a preview in my mind, word for word, of what they subsequently said out loud. I got up and went back to my desk.

Separating the Signal from the Noise

The chiropractor had talked about how, when he first started the chiropractic energy work, people were dropping things around him, in stores and such. That opened my eyes to what I had observed in previous episodes. It was clear that one needed to strive to keep energy responses coming from right action. *Right action* is a term that is used in Eastern philosophies to describe having the right motives in your thoughts and actions.

In the hospital I had noticed other people struggling with magical thinking. One patient confided in me that when the nurse scratched her nose, it meant something. To me it meant that she was lost in her magical thinking.

Other patients were plagued with situations such as getting on the subway and finding everyone looked familiar. John, who described this unnerving event, said at another time that everyone seemed to be signalling him.

At this point, I took my right arm and waved it slowly behind the back of my head while asking, "What sort of signals are you getting?"

He laughed for about five minutes as a result. I often used humour internally and with others.

John attempted suicide by running a car in closed garage. Instead of dying, he lost his short-term memory.

After that, I didn't talk to him for a long time. I happened to be outside his apartment building one Saturday morning with Eric and, on a whim, decided to visit him. He was in the final stages of dying from complications of some sort and died the next day. His mother called me and mentioned how surprised and pleased he was to see me and asked if I would attend his funeral. Of course I did.

Mike was staying for free, but had to put up with a lot. It's not easy living with, or even being around, someone with inner turmoil. At one point I got so involved with the inner battle that I literally punched my own jaw. I described this to Mike, and he sort of walked through the motions himself to see if it was even possible.

Mike Crosses the Pond

Eric and I would go with Mike to soccer games. Even though he was in his fifties, Mike and a group of friends were in a very competitive league. They let me play a bit, but the inner conversation would interfere with my ability to play.

Mike left after a few months to go back to England. Eric and I were sad to see him go. I contacted him once by phone, but even though he had my number, he never tried to contact me.

Energy Work

MY THOUGHTS AND ENERGY EXPERIENCES GOT WORSE. I remember asking my friend from Montreal and his live-in girlfriend if they would take Eric. They said they could take him to ball games or other such things, but weren't about to step in.

I asked my mother if she would come from Montreal and live with us, but she recognized that it would pull her down rather than help me.

I did make a friend within the chiropractic circle. She was a massage therapist, although she wasn't practicing at this point. Eric and I hit it off with her. She and I would do energy work together. She would get me on her portable adjustment table and run her hands above my body, checking for heat levels and blending the energy.

Our friendship lasted a number of years. She would try to do energy work on me while I was frantic. At one point, I was at her place, north of Toronto. My thinking was choppy and frenetic. She got me on the massage table and tried to get a hold of my energy and slow it down, to no avail. I recall going for a walk around the block with her. I had bursts of energy over and over in my head as we walked. It was as if part of me was trying to kill me off.

The next day we drove to the chiropractor. He put me on a table, and I felt a release. He exclaimed that I had released an entity that filled the room.

One problem I had with his services was he was Catholic, and a couple of times he brought me into a room and seemed to be casting out demons in Christ's name. I don't think someone in a bipolar condition should be too caught up in good and evil. The first time he did this, I got very religious for a time. I felt evil stalking me. I would see the number 666 on license plates or other places, and that would become meaningful.

I got a bit of an antidote when playing piano a while later at a lodge in Hamilton. The waiter was very upset because certain numbers that he felt were meaningful and evil kept coming up on the bills. It helped to see my own problem projected out in someone else, and this lessened my own concern. It was a bit of a synchronistic event to see this guy struggle with the symbolism behind everyday numbers.

Meanwhile, on a daily basis, I was in deep distress. At one point, I went to Ashbridges Bay on Lake Ontario in January. The thoughts had reached a frenzy and stayed that way for days, with no letup. The thoughts were screaming at me to jump into the lake. So I did. I swam in a circle and decided it was not a good day to die. Or at least it wasn't good weather for it. So I got out, and with ice forming all over my winter coat and pants, I made my way back home with the stream of crazy thoughts taunting me.

I couldn't find my house keys, so I kicked in the back door. I took a bath as my energy went sky high and then compressed down on top of me over and over.

It took a while to reconcile my condition in terms of bipolarity, in which good and evil is a pair of opposites.

At one point I became convinced I needed to drive out the demons in my mind. I needed to become like an exorcist. I remember, right after deciding this, being in the local park with a couple of other people and dogs around. I commanded my dog to heel.

The guy beside me said, "Spoken like a true exorcist."

I took this as a firm indicator that I was right and that I needed to drive out my demons. That never happened. It was bad advice. One strong lesson I have learned is you can manifest your misconceptions, just as you can get beneficial direction, in subtle ways.

In one of the books I read, there was a section that suggested that when there is a separation of the parts of the personality, and a part is not blended with the rest, a part of you must die. I may have misinterpreted this. I think the author meant the relationship of a part of your personality to the rest must change. But I spent a lot of time thinking that I was supposed to kill off a part of myself, which probably did more damage than good.

Since then I have taken to a Chinese saying that in order to kill a beast, you must first make it pretty. My version is that in order to *tame* a beast, you must first make it pretty.

Luckily I was doing a lot of reading. I was into the poetry of Rumi:

> Beyond wrongdoing and rightdoing, there is a field, I'll meet you there.

I've gone from overwhelming bipolarities to this field. It's wonderful and sustaining. I consider it to be oceanic.

My own belief system includes God, but I don't believe in hell. As Joseph Campbell puts it:

> The problem with hell is that the fire doesn't consume you. The fires of transformation do.

Rumi was a thirteenth-century Persian poet who believed in spiritual evolution. Another of his poems elaborates this belief:

> I died as a mineral and became a plant,
> I died as plant and rose to animal,
> I died as animal and I was Man.
> Why should I fear? When was I less by dying?
> Yet once more I shall die as Man, to soar
> With angels bless'd; but even from angelhood
> I must pass on: all except God doth perish.
> When I have sacrificed my angel-soul,
> I shall become what no mind e'er conceived.
> Oh, let me not exist! for Non-existence
> Proclaims in organ tones,
> To Him we shall return.
> Generation after generation lies down, defeated, they think,
> but they're like a woman underneath a man, circling him.

One molecule-mate-second thinking of God's reversal of
comfort
and pain is better than any attending ritual. That splinter
of intelligence is substance.
The fire and water themselves:
Accidental, done with mirrors.

My own belief system is along the same lines. Perhaps we have one life as
a human as Rumi seems to suggest. Or maybe we're here to learn lessons,
and until we get it right, we come back, under the big sky, with the unre-
solved wishes and fears to be addressed once more.

A Different Hospital

I floundered at the company where I continued to show up for work.
There came a point where I could no longer go to work. I could no longer
sleep. I was lost in the signals.

I was brought to Wellesley Hospital, the same hospital where my
father died. I was fascinated by the patterns on the wall in an isolated
room in Emergency. A nurse sat down beside me and gave me some
medication. I woke up realizing I was watching and trying to make
sense of the patterns on a curtain in the close observation room on
the psychiatric floor. My conscious awareness was enough to break the
fascination.

My house was a mess. The whole family got involved this time, as no
one knew where Eric was. He had taken change from my chest of drawers
and taken the streetcar to school. My family shared the responsibility of
providing food and shelter for Eric until I recovered.

I had a different hospital experience. The psychiatrist was proud to
say that the walls were grey and that this was beneficial. The reasoning
for this escapes me. I recovered to a certain extent, but I felt heavy and
broken.

The doctor wanted me to go back to work and phoned and arranged
it. As soon as I got there, I was in a state of anxiety. I could barely follow a conversation. My boss took me aside and told me that he had to
let me go.

So I went back to the hospital. I was more relaxed and okay there. I was released after a few more weeks. There wasn't a lot of therapy going on. I was out and back to looking for a job.

The medication I was put on at Wellesley was debilitating. A horrible cocktail of drugs that affected my movements. I went to my family doctor and got put back on lithium.

Someone from the men's group was making good money contracting through a high-end consulting company. I spoke to his boss and got a position.

On the second day of work, I felt my fragile state slip into an episode. They noticed that I was very quiet. While taking minutes for a meeting, it was noticed that I could type very fast. One of the consultants decided that I would be useful as a scribe during their meetings. It involved listening to what was going on in the room and typing. I was good at that.

The head consultant decided to use me in another set of meetings. But this time he wanted me to type only what he wrote on the flip chart. It was a useless thing to do. I should have told him that I could do that after the meeting and let me capture the conversation as I did the first time, but I was barely holding on and went along with this.

I had gone to a seminar years before about a mind control method, something called Silva Mind Control, which I haven't heard anything about in the past twenty-five years. They stated that they were able to go without glasses because their mind could adjust and their vision would be fine. So I started going without glasses. I had trouble seeing detail in the distance, but my eyesight was good enough for most things.

As years went by, my eyes got worse. I tried to read what was being captured on the flip charts. I couldn't do it. It was a bit of a scandal, as I was told not to come back until I had a pair of glasses. So I got the glasses and was able to continue—but not for long. They laid me off soon afterward. I was one of the walking wounded the whole time I was there.

The Epiphany

I SPENT A LOT OF TIME COMING to grips with my thinking and what my life was about. My mind was a whirlwind. I was quite aware of the synchronicity and symbolism around me. My distant past seemed to open up, and events that were years apart seemed to have a sense of synchronicity. This seemed beyond what Carl Jung had written about.

One example was something that happened in grade one. I was in the class listening to the teacher read *The Little Engine that Could*. She pointed to the driver and said that he was the engineer. I blurted out that my father was an engineer. She asked if he was that type of engineer, and I said yes.

So I went home and asked my father what kind of engineer he was. He announced that he was a civil engineer. I was crestfallen. I don't know why it bothered me so much that he didn't say he was a train engineer. It was a year later when I went to the teacher and told her my father wasn't a train engineer. Of course, this was not a issue for her and she was very kind as she reassured me about it.

I forgot about it.

Years later, my parents divorced, and my mother married a train engineer.

On the surface, this is just a coincidence. But it was a meaningful coincidence for me. I didn't recognize the coincidence at first. It came to me in the middle of a bipolar episode when I was in my late thirties.

Another event that became linked at this time was a trip I took with my father. I was about twelve years old, and my father was going to Northern Quebec, to a small airport. My father was the construction engineer for building runways. This was the one and only father-son trip we had. My father sat in the back of the small Beechcraft Baron, and I sat in the copilot's seat. At one point in the trip, the pilot told me I could take control of the steering wheel. Every move I made would cause the plane to move. I was nervous and asked the pilot to take back the controls.

He remarked, "That's funny. Most boys enjoy flying the plane."

I was very embarrassed in front of my father.

About ten years later, I went to a county fair just before university started. They had free flight lesson coupons. I took one. The next weekend I went to the airport and had my lesson. After takeoff, the pilot let me take control of the steering wheel. I followed the ground and flew over the house I was living in. Then I flew the plane to the university grounds. All of a sudden, another plane was right in front of us and veered away with about twenty feet between us. It was almost a head on collision. I calmly asked the pilot if we were at the right altitude. He radioed the tower, stated that we were where we should be, and we finished our flight. I was calm the whole time. I had a sense of well-being when I left the airport.

My calmness flying the plane, even during a potential midflight collision, was the karmic antidote to the flight with my father.

But it wasn't until this moment that I connected the two events. Since this time I look for events that have a synchronistic nature. They are much more apparent when I am on shaky ground. They seem rather mundane when I am on firm ground.

I may not have recognized any synchronistic events without having read all kinds of philosophy books and undergone the chiropractic and medical care. I never would have read these books without having a condition that drove me to keep looking for a cure. It has been said that an unexamined life is not worth living. In this context, my life has certainly been worth living.

I WAS WALKING THE DOG WITH the usual rough and very active energy coursing through my body. It had been going on for months, with very little break. I had a notion that there might be something I could do by surrendering to the energy.

As I walked along, I would feel the energy in my gut. I would picture the other side, where the energy was pushing against in my mind and body. I would be at one with the other side and soften up and let the rough energy penetrate.

I found an analogy to yin and yang energy from Chinese and other Eastern philosophies. I started to experience a sense of ecstasy as the energies melded. This was especially true in my abdomen.

It didn't stop the split in my thinking, where there was a sense of two or more thought processes going on at the same time, vying for supremacy, yet not responding to any dialogue with what I considered my regular thoughts.

Once my mind speeds up, there's nowhere to hide. Sleep gets very difficult, which became both a symptom and a cause of the internal distress.

I went to a friend's cottage outside of Ottawa. My body language was such that my hands were handcuffed as the thinking storm continued during the car ride there.

That evening in the cottage, I went to bed and instead of sleeping, I went back into yielding to the yin and yang. I spent the night surfing the energy, which felt very, very good. The next morning, the doublethink was still there, quick to assert itself, and the mind storm continued.

There's a poem of Rumi's that describes the yin and yang of my experience quite well:

God's presence is there in front of me, a fire on the left,
a lovely stream on the right.
One group walks toward the fire, *into* the fire, another
toward the sweet flowing water.
No one knows which are blessed and which not.
Whoever walks into the fire appears suddenly in the stream.
A head goes under on the water surface, that head
pokes out of the fire.
Most people guard against going into the fire,
and so end up in it.
Those who love the water of pleasure and make it their devotion
are cheated with this reversal.
The trickery goes further.
The voice of the fire tells the *truth,* saying *I am not fire.*
I am fountainhead. Come into me and don't mind the sparks.
If you are a friend of God, fire is your water.
You should wish to have a hundred thousand sets of mothwings,
so you could burn them away, one set a night.
The moth sees light and goes into fire. You should see fire
and go toward light. Fire is what of God is world-consuming.
Water, world-protecting.
Somehow each gives the appearance of the other. To these eyes
you have now what looks like water burns.
What looks like fire is a great relief to be inside.
You've seen a magician make a bowl of rice
seem a dish full of tiny live worms.
Before an assembly with one breath he made the floor swarm
with scorpions that weren't there.
How much more amazing God's tricks.

What I had discovered walking the dog, and continued with at my friend's cottage, became a method of going into the fire and landing up in the water. I could lie in bed and do this yin-yang thing. But it still was not a cure for my condition.

The following Tuesday I went to the men's group. The Welsh co-leader was into energy work, as this was what the whole group was about. He looked over at me and said that he could see that I was loving myself, that my energy showed that. I mentioned this to a First Nations fellow whom I was giving a drive home. He agreed. I asked what the energy was.

He said, as a matter of fact, "Love."

Pairs of Opposites

Joseph Campbell quoted Nietzsche and wrote:

> Goethe says, "Everything temporal is but a metaphor." Nietzsche says, "Everything is but a metaphor." They are saying the same thing. "Everything" includes God, heaven, hell, the whole works. So as long as you are living to get to heaven you won't find that still place. One has to go beyond the pair of opposites to find the real source.

To someone with bipolar disorder, it is interesting to hear about going beyond pairs of opposites. It has a tangible quality about it. I've been there. I felt like an accidental tourist into ways that very few sages and scholars attained although many ways were attempted.

Big Company

While feeling relatively normal, I went on some interviews and was offered a position at an international company. I went in as a project leader and struggled with my condition on and off. I had a fairly easy project, and contract staff to develop it.

I was hired by a guy who was making considerable funds with software he wrote and sold on a website. He wanted me to do the day-to-day activities while he and a colleague maintained another product and he would be free to tend to his website customers.

There was a contract person from Russia who was learning English. I taught him how to model computer systems, for which he was very grateful. I hired another person, and a summer student wunderkind returned on a co-op assignment to complete my development group.

We would play ping-pong at noon, and as long as the pressure was off, I was doing okay. I was still on lithium and nothing else.

I noticed that the senior manager had nothing to do with the project and my manager focused more on another, bigger project. Anytime I had a meeting or encounter with management, I would be anxious. But I had once again put together a good team, and we produced an excellent accounting software product.

My manager appreciated my work. His own work was considered only adequate in a review, and in a political manoeuvre, he landed up as a senior manager in another department.

There were layoffs. I was kept, but the guy who brought me in was let go to play with his website on his own time. He was very sore about this.

The software my team built was well received. However, with cutbacks, it was soon to be discontinued. My senior manager was very happy to see it taken out of service. I don't understand why he felt this way.

The person who came in as a replacement project manager of our group did not appreciate me. At this point I was involved with potential year 2000 date issues for an existing system. I was somewhat manic, which meant I was sort of childlike. He didn't see me as a project leader. We met for my review, and I was relegated to working on first-line support for the other product that they had been building. I was to report to another project leader, which was a big loss of face. I was happy to hang on to my job though, as my thinking was interrupted constantly, and I was not able to concentrate and build an understanding of the software.

Black Swans

There was a walking path on the side the company building in Brampton.

On the path, there was a pool with ducks and two black swans. The swans came from Australia. They were named Thelma and Louise.

Years later I read a book about black swans. In trading circles a black swan is an improbable event where a stock or other trading instrument takes a huge dive.

The original idea about the swans was that it was considered at one time that all swans were white. That was before they discovered Australia. It took only one black swan to refute the theory.

I find it ironic that this company bought two black swans and named them after a movie ending with Thelma and Louise going for a big dive off the Grand Canyon.

Their stock went from over one hundred dollars to penny stock in a very short period of time. I had been buying stock on payroll for years. Like a lot of people, I lost a lot of money.

Some coincidence, those swans.

Chiropractic Gates

I WAS SEEING A DIFFERENT CHIROPRACTOR, who was also a follower of the first chiropractor's process. She wasn't having much luck getting me out of stuck positions, but saw that I was aware of the collective consciousness and synchronistic events. She decided that I was a good candidate to meet the founder at one of his gates. A *gate* was the term for a weekend intensive where a number of chiropractors would perform energy work on a number of "practice members" in a hotel seminar room.

I went to see the founder at a gate in Denver. Beforehand he phoned me and expressed concern because he had not had much success with people with bipolar disorder. I explained that I had a pretty strong internal witness, and I was enrolled. The internal witness is my way of saying that I have a calm place inside that observes what is going on and the state of my condition. It is what has sustained me during psychosis and enabled me to continue to function and work.

There was a snowstorm when I was to fly to Denver. Flights were being cancelled, but I had the sense that I was going to make it there regardless. While other people going to the same destination were delayed or had their flights cancelled, my trip went like clockwork.

I was in relatively okay shape but the founder noticed something obvious to him about my energy situation and made a point of doing adjustments on me personally.

I had been on lithium for years. I recalled the men's group and how medication might be an impediment to really getting into this life-changing opportunity. I decided to go off the lithium and told the founder so. That called for high fives. But he did not coach me to go off the medication.

So he pronounced me to be "in the flow" after the last adjustment. He had two other gates planned in the near future, an intensive one in Sicily

79

or thereabouts and a double weekend in Como, Italy. He cautioned me that the Sicily gate would be too intense for me, so I signed up for Como.

The time between the Denver and the Como gates was a rollicking time. I was in the flow, alright. I was seeing patterns everywhere. I was a mess. I continued to go to work. There were orange decorative spots at various places on the floor at work. I started navigating by the colour orange.

I would come home from work and immediately go upstairs and have a bath while reading self-help and philosophy books. I remember reading Carl Jung at lunchtime. The concept of synchronicity seemed so obvious.

I had trouble sitting in an office because it appeared that my thoughts had a strong influence on the people around me, and my thoughts were playing cat and mouse with me. Various polarities appeared to be happening both internally and within the room.

I would sit at my desk and feel my inner turmoil and hear the sounds in the room ebbing and flowing in unison. I was in the flow, but I was not grounded.

Como, Italy

I considered cancelling the trip to Como as my condition was so bad. I talked to a lady recommended by my current chiropractor. She was considered to be psychic. She told me that I was very psychic and my energy was either shut off or all over the room. She told me to go soft and let whatever was taking place happen. She said something about being like a dinosaur that was evolving, whatever that meant. I took her literally.

So I went to Como. The airport was interesting in that I was very aware of a couple and their child and the energy between them. It was as though we were underwater and you could sense the water currents after each movement of the hand or whatever. Once again, the phenomenon was *oceanic*.

This concept of oceanic was introduced by Romain Rolland and popularized by Freud:

> It is a sensation of an indissoluble bond, as of being connected with the external world in its integral form...The "oceanic

feeling" described as a oneness with the world or a limitless-
ness is simply a description of the feeling the infant has before it
learns there are other persons in the world. On the contrary, the
oceanic feeling, the sense of wonder, leads people to a humble
awareness of Truth, with some sense of the human ego's relative
size and importance in the whole universe. This is a feeling that
can only be experienced in totality and not without conscious
awareness and certainty.

The actual plane ride wasn't oceanic. It was terrifying. I felt my thoughts
were connected to the turbulence. I was afraid of my thinking and worried
about the plane crashing. The lady who sat next to me said her name, which
I don't recall, but it was unusual. She said it meant "peace and quiet."

When we got off the plane in Milan, the airport was spotless and col-
ourful. The lady asked me if I could appreciate how peaceful the airport
was. We walked to the bus stops. She was going downtown. I wandered
away and came across a bus for Como. It dropped me off in the village. I
got a lift from someone to the Como Hotel, but it was the wrong one. So
I took my suitcase and walked out of town in a random direction. I found
the Grand Hotel of Como, and it was the right one.

I was early, as usual. A guy who played guitar during the first gate in
Denver was there. He also played beautiful piano, and we both played the
grand piano in the dining area. As usual when in a fragile state, I played
quite eloquently.

I had a room with marble floors. I found my mind fascinated by the
cracks in the floor, making patterns and finding esoteric meanings for
them. My mind was going a mile a minute.

When I met up with the founder, he remarked that my energy was
much better now. It wasn't. It was much worse than when I was in Denver.

He did a number of chiropractic entrainments (the word they started
using for adjustments). He noticed when I would get up and walk that my
breath and movement were matched. He remarked positively on that. I
noticed as I walked around that people would start to groan and move
around. I seem to have an effect on the room. Since one of the principle

purposes of entrainments was to get into your condition and live through it, I may have been doing people a favour, to the extent I was involved.

There were five days between the gates in Como. I was alone and in a very fragile state. I went to Milan. I had to relinquish my passport to the hotelkeeper. I went for a walk in the evening and came across a small restaurant. There was a very pretty girl serving pizza. An older, well-dressed, muscular man appeared to own the restaurant. He saw me looking at the girl and asked disingenuously if I liked her. I said she seemed fine. He left me alone.

Since my energy was all over the map, and my mind jumpy, I got the sense that I could send some energy to this girl. So I did. She stopped in mid-step and looked bothered. She seemed to recognize at some level what I had done.

I paid and left. I stumbled around town without finding my hotel. I happened past the same restaurant again and, being a fool, went in. I sat with the waitress as she prepared paperwork at the end of the evening. I ordered a bottle of water. I behaved myself. But the well-dressed, muscular guy had it in for me. His English wasn't great, so he brought an egg from the kitchen and showed it to me, indicating that I was like that. I didn't know what he meant.

He said, "Sympatico," which to me was the name of an Internet service provider. I didn't know what he meant.

He drew a fish on a piece of paper with bars in front of it. I had really gotten his attention. Two ladies sat down at the next table. A guy came in selling flowers. I bought some and gave them to the two ladies. The muscular guy was still on my case. He showed me a card in his wallet. The card had the title Marco Polo. That was supposed to mean something to me. I thought it was probably an indication that he was connected with the Italian police, or maybe the Mafia, or both. The two ladies, the waitress, and the muscular guy got up to leave. He told me to leave too. I indicated that I was staying until I finished my water. They left together.

I managed to find the small hotel I was staying at. I phoned home and talked to my son. He expressed to his mother that I was really in bad shape.

I was sleeping okay. Without sleep, I have no means of recuperation. I continued my journey in Northern Italy. I found a hotel in the country that was inexpensive and elegant. I put my American Express money in a pair of pants where I thought it would be safe. Half a day later, I couldn't find it. I spent an hour with the concierge trying to find the number to call to contact American Express to cancel the cheques. He wouldn't let me use the Internet. I found that if I walked onto the carpet, he would move a certain way, and if I walked to the corner, he would move differently. I finally gave up and went to bed. When I woke up in the morning, I put my hand in my pants and found my cheques.

There was a small park near this hotel that had a lot of garbage on the ground. I found I could get my mind to agree on something. Picking up and separating the garbage was an activity that seemed to appease my mind. I spent about an hour at this.

It's too bad I was so pre-occupied as the country side was beautiful. I'd like to go back there some day.

I was able to limp through the week. I made my way back to Como, and the weather and lake were beautiful. I bought a disposable camera. I took dozens of pictures. Somehow the pictures seemed to have deep symbolic meaning. I kept going back to the store and bought camera after camera. I found a very small airport with one or two water planes. This seemed terribly meaningful, and I took plenty of pictures.

Somehow I got it in my head that Italy had solved the pollution problem. There was moss growing between the rail tracks. Technology and ecology seemed to have come together. I came to the conclusion that the positioning of the highways was curing pollution. I also found meaning in the colour of cars and their ordering on highways.

While walking to the Grand Hotel, I came across a gas station and bought all their atlases. I was haemorrhaging money.

The second weekend was more frenetic than the first. The seating arrangement at the start of the sessions seemed meaningful. A lady in the front row seemed to be aligned with me. I decided that I was to marry her. Another guy seemed like a genuinely decent guy, the type I would want for a friend.

I announced to the girl that we were supposed to marry. She was puz-
zled, and concerned for me. She met me by the piano, and I played a bit
while she talked. She tried successfully to reason with me. I was coming
down from the extreme manic condition I was in. I played beautifully and
could feel strong energy flowing from my hands.

She pointed at my hands and said, "What do you think that is?"

I said, "Love."

She was a great singer and sang for me. I admitted as we parted that I
didn't know why I considered marrying her, but that I was having a terrible time and finding meanings that were spurious.

I got through the second weekend with little enthusiasm.

The last dinner at the Grand Hotel of Como was with the founder and
other staff. He repeated the sentiment that my movements matched my
breath. To this day, when I think of it, I try to match my movements to
my breath.

I shared a taxi back to the airport with three chiropractors. They asked
if I was DC, meaning a licensed chiropractor. I said I was AC, Air Canada.
They laughed. As we approached the airport, my anxiety level rose. I had
had such a bad flight there. They seemed to pick up on that, and one of
them noticed some guy-wires for a roof. He commented that it looked like
a big clamp holding everything together. I took that as reassuring.

I was okay for the trip back. I got talking to an opera singer who
seemed to pick up on my unspoken nuances, and we had a nice time. It
was a much better flight back.

I wrote a long e-mail to the founder. It was a very manic composition.
The last time I saw him was to pay fifty dollars for the privilege of hearing
him speak. I went up to talk to him, and he said, "Oh you're the one who
wrote that long e-mail," then turned to talk to someone else.

I went back on lithium.

I really think he's on to something, but it no longer works for me. It
might be because I'm on medication. But I'll take medication and memories of energy states over psychosis and energy phenomena.

Back to Work

I CONTINUED TO FLOAT IN AND OUT OF EPISODES. There was someone who I was asked to mentor when he first started. We became pretty good friends for a while. I went a little manic and came up with some words that I enjoyed and wished to share. This guy expressed that he lost respect for me. I told him that I was manic-depressive and couldn't always help myself. That didn't help.

Mental illness is not a solid defense in most scenarios. It is best kept a secret. There are some notable exceptions of famous people who are known to be bipolar and may actually be more respected for having coped with their condition.

I got a book from a doctor I had a lot of respect for. I went in a very agitated state, wondering how I was going to continue at work and support my son and keep a roof over his head. She closed the door and announced that she was manic-depressive. I would have never guessed. I imagine there are people who know me who would have never guessed. She loaned me *An Unquiet Mind* to read. I read it and then bought my own copy. I have read it many times.

I also noticed a book on her bookshelf about people and patterns. She let me borrow that one as well. I found it fascinating, as it showed a picture of a man, and a woman, with a dog on her shoulder. It talked about how energy is shared between people as they navigate the ebbs and flows of energy in the world. Although it was a medical text, I found this book helped me understand the energy levels I had experienced.

My son was at home most of the time, on the computer. We had a very stilted relationship. He would express to his mother how angry he was when I got sick.

His mother seemed to have stabilized. She was living with this guy in an apartment. He had received a large inheritance, but had a gambling habit. She could finish a case of twenty-four beers in an evening and look for more.

Eric had trouble attending school. He spent most of his time playing role-playing games on the computer. He would play late at night and into the morning, sleep in, eat, and play some more. I finally got him enrolled in a school for troubled children, where his attendance improved.

His last two years of high school were stellar. He got himself enrolled in a regular high school and then a specialized gifted high school. He was at the top of the class and got a scholarship for university.

Meanwhile, I had the sense that I was sinking once again into psychosis. It got very intense. I had a friend coming over to help me paint the house. She looked me over and suggested we go for a walk around the block. I felt like a condemned man taking his last walk. She told Eric that he needed to get me into the hospital.

Eric told me to lie on his bed and called a family member. My friend left. I had the sensation that the furnace was getting louder and louder. I was afraid it was going to explode unless I shifted my position, which I did over and over.

Help arrived and I was driven to Wellesley Hospital. But it was closed for good. It was being torn down, grey walls and all. So we went to St. Mike's.

St. Mike's

I DIDN'T FEEL THE USUAL SURGE OF ANGER when going into the hospital. I entered in an agitated state. When I got into the swing, it seemed that the attendants and nurses were not in great shape themselves.

I remember watching a movie, *A Fish Called Wanda*, which I had originally watched a decade earlier. I originally found it hilarious. It was one of the funniest movies I recalled seeing. In the hospital, I watched it with a very depressed man. We agreed that the movie was quite sad. Watching a hockey game was like watching zombies lurch all over the ice.

I felt like I was in a state of limbo. I had a sense of synchronicity, but I just felt beyond life. I was put on a new medication this time, olanzapine. I basically went through the paces at the hospital and didn't feel very well. I met with the doctor and said that I was okay, although I wasn't, and was released. He didn't write me a prescription for olanzapine because he didn't think it was a good long-term medication. One of the side effects listed was tardive dyskinesia—involuntary movements of the mouth, tongue, jaw, or eyelids. That side effect appears on a number of medications that I have found. The list of side effects for most medications is not for the faint of heart.

I went back to work, but didn't last long. I went back in a very agitated state and phoned my family doctor. I asked her which hospital I should go to, and she suggested a psychiatric hospital. I had always gone to general hospitals. So I took her advice and took the streetcar there. I was in the waiting room with my *An Unquiet Mind* book to read once more. After a while they announced that they were full and the only hospital available was St. Mike's.

I was impressed with the irony that, of all the hospitals around, the only one available was the one I had left prematurely. I was to go back and continue the treatment I hadn't finished at St. Mike's.

There's an iconic statue in this hospital that shows an angel with a raised sword, and dark matter under her feet. I took it to mean that in order to be in the light, you have to pin down your shadow. Sort of like Jesus saying, "Get thee behind me, Satan." I wasn't really interested in being the light, but I had experience with the bipolarity of darkness and light. "The closer to the light, the longer the shadow" comes to mind.

So I was back on the ward and back on olanzapine. This was the last time I was hospitalized to the present day, ten years later.

When I got out, I contacted my psychiatric doctor, and he agreed that olanzapine was a good drug to be on. I insisted on remaining on lithium, and he noted that there was a lot of research indicating the combination of the two drugs worked very well.

He is a medicine man. He had a little statue of Buddha that I asked about. He said a patient had given it to him and he had little idea what Buddha represented. I thought that all major religions and philosophies should be required reading for a psychiatrist. But he is a good doctor, he has a lot of compassion, and I continue to get treatment from him.

Out of Work

I WAS LAID OFF AROUND 2002. It was a bad time to look for a job. I met a fellow who said I could get work in a placement agency firm he was a partner in. So I got involved.

I kept my hand in on computer work. With two partners, I started a company to get websites up and running.

The head-hunting job was straight commission. The boss sat in his office, but the main guy was a talented recruiter who ran the floor. He left under sudden circumstance and took most of the floor with him. I made a little money, left for another firm, and never received the bulk of the funds I earned.

The second firm I worked for was straight head-hunting: call up a company and fib your way into getting names of potential candidates. I couldn't stand it and left.

I got the website company off the ground. The other two partners provided some of the funds while I figured out how to use some third-party software to jump-start building the sites. Creating sites turned out to be easy; making money was pretty much impossible. I learned a lot about sourcing and developing associations with manufacturing companies to be an additional site offering their products. I also learned something about search engine optimization.

I got a second job at a university doing surveys. It was very similar to telemarketing, and I did not enjoy it.

My spending was very frugal, but I was losing money every month.

I got onto an internet dating service. I called it *51 First Dates*, like the movie, but instead with a different woman every time.

I met one lady whom I found easy to talk to. She was in computer contracting. She was very helpful, saying that I needed to get back into mainstream computer work. She helped me piece my career together. We landed up getting married a year later.

I was interested in modelling systems, and had experience with it in the past, so she had me read up on it. Sure enough, one of the banks was looking for a modeller, and I found a position as a business analyst, doing modelling.

Over the years, I have developed a more pronounced tremour in my hands. It is barely discernible when I am relaxed, but my hands flutter like birds when I am under stress. Wherever I work, someone always seems to comment on it.

I don't smoke or drink. I quit years ago. I probably shook more because I take lithium. But I think it was also because I have gone through so much and my nervous system is affected.

I was preparing for a meeting. My preparation involved running through and tracing exactly what steps the software was to perform. It was pages and pages of steps and numbers. I was explaining it to the project manager. My hands shook so much that I could barely turn the pages. He was stymied as to what I was trying to do and asked who had told me to do this. I said that he did. He said that the business folks were not going to be able to follow it in Monday's meeting. I felt exposed and afraid of losing my job.

I spent the weekend with my fiancée, showing her what I wrote and wondering what I was going to do with it. My energy was a mess. It was nowhere near the bipolarities of the past, but it was the worse condition that she had seen me in.

She took my raw data and put it together in summary form in a spread-sheet. It was great. Although my hands were so shaky in the meeting that I could barely turn the page, I walked through the process and asked if there were any questions. There were none. The project manager nodded at me, as if to say, *"Good job."*

Manifest Misconceptions

THE ABILITY OF THE MIND TO MAKE connections is a double-edged sword. When someone is in a psychotic state, they start to manifest their beliefs, fears, and suspicions. Not every connection is accurate or healthy. If not grounded, they can get lost. They cannot separate the signal from the noise. The psychiatric term is *magical thinking*.

Magical thinking is described in the article by Lisa Fritscher in an About.com guide:

> Magical thinking is a clinical term used to describe a wide variety of nonscientific and sometimes irrational beliefs. These beliefs are generally centered on correlations between events.

This is very true of people under mental duress. They can make conclusions as to what their own mind means when making connections. They can get on a wrong tack about it.

One thing that they may have going for them is the sense of a witness I described earlier, the inner observer that doesn't fall into the thinking traps that form and reform throughout the illness. The inner observer can refuse to buy into it even as the mind is fascinated and continues to fall into it. The observer can also recognize when the connection being made is valid.

Frogs All Over the Place

Toward the end of Dr. J's career, she started to collect frogs. There were velvet cloth frogs, ceramic frogs, all types. Frogs were all over her office. It seemed to me, upon reflection, that the growing number of frogs represented all the frogs she kissed that didn't turn into princes.

Recently I met another therapist who had on display a ceramic frog. When asked about it, she proclaimed that it was important because it was the only creature that could go in only one direction; it couldn't go backward.

I mentioned my interpretation, and she laughed and said, "That too!"

On my Dharma

SINCE MARRIAGE, I HAVE CONTINUED TO CONTRACT in the computer field. I still have my ups and downs. I stay on olanzapine and lithium. I also use sleeping pills when necessary. When I am over-stressed at work, my sleep suffers. The sleeping medication, Zopiclone, is nonaddictive and doesn't lose it potency with use. I usually don't need it.

Synchronicity

I continue to be fascinated by synchronicity and energy work. I have tried various chiropractors, but found that the light touch practitioners no longer have an effect on me. So I sometimes see a regular chiropractor who can physically move my spine.

I look for examples of synchronicity. They are generally of the garden variety. Here are a few:

- My wife is fed up with my backseat driving and tells me so. A few minutes later, a lady tries to pass her on the right and she would have hit her if I hadn't yelled at her about it.
- I made a point of looking for synchronicity while shopping for non-alcoholic wine. The wine brand was "Carl Jung." Sort of a cosmic joke.

So I'm not finding earth-shaking examples, but it helps to try to salvage some of the experiences of the past with my everyday life of today.

Joseph Campbell wrote about when you are close to enlightenment, synchronicity grows stronger. I find the opposite is true but if you persist in looking for synchronicity, you can find it.

Energy Work

More interesting is the energy play that I'm finding.

I had a project manager while working at a bank. I wasn't getting along with her too well, and my energy was a bit rough. I was walking along a corridor from the bathroom, when she turned the corner, approaching me from the other way. I said hi, but my energy surged. She kept walking, bent over, and sort of leaned against the wall going by me.

Another time I was in a much softer energy state. In this state, my eyes go soft, and I find I am focused on the expressions on people's faces. The same project manager was very friendly and touched me on the shoulder as we spoke. It was entirely a different energy and response. I try to be in this state as much as possible.

When I am in a state where my body electric is very active, I lie down on my back and let the rough energy penetrate the calm areas. This is the yin-yang effect described earlier.

Quantum Physics

I'm interested in the findings of quantum physics. They talk about pairs of opposites (entanglements) and how, by observing a quantum event, one can "collapse" probable outcomes into a finite event.

The idea that quantum events only occur at the quantum level has been, and is being, challenged.

Back when quantum physics were first being discussed, Schrödinger wrote about how the quantum-level activities could have an effect on the macro level. His story about a cat being alive and dead according to a quantum event is famous. There are other more recent examples of quantum events determined within day-to-day life.

The Act of Observation

I like to think that the quantum finding that the act of observing changes what is being observed applies at the macro level. More than just the act of observing, the interpretation and wished-for outcome has an effect on what is observed now or in the future. This is similar to praying.

I still go into fragile states, but with the faith that the medicine will prevent me from straying too far into an episode. In some ways I look forward to a bit of shaky ground. My eyes go soft; I play beautiful piano.

Sigmund Freud & Eric Berne

FREUD DEVELOPED A PSYCHODYNAMIC model that describes the superego, ego, and id. Eric Berne further developed this into a transactional analysis model where there is a corresponding parent, adult, and child. He describes how communication can be carried out between one person's parent and another person's parent, or adult to adult, or child to child. Communication is also smooth when one's parent talks to another's child and the other person responds from the child perspective back to the first person's parent. Trouble brews when there is a crossed transaction. For instance, a person communicates from his parent to the other's child, while the other person responds from his parent.

Berne describes games that people play without awareness or with some awareness. His book *Games People Play* became a best seller. While it comes across to me as a condemnation, I find it fascinating that there is unconscious or semiconscious communication that is very inventive. It reminds me of the multiple levels of communication I have witnessed along the way. I have found that games are played within a person as well as between people.

In many of the books I have read, there is an emphasis on staying alert in the present moment. I find that being in the present moment keeps me from getting involved with game playing.

What interests me also is the concept that a person with bipolar disorder oscillates between having a parent and adult functioning with a blocked child, and when in an alternate state the person has an adult and child active, while the parent is blocked. This resonates with me at a deep level.

Acceptance of the Condition

JOSEPH CAMPBELL AND OTHERS HAVE WRITTEN about creating a hero's story for one's life. My wife and a few friends have supported me in turning my story of weakness and cowardliness into this story of myself as a hero, continuing an epic journey.

Everybody has the opportunity to position themselves as a hero. Life changes magically when you do. Selective memories of the past change accordingly. Examples of personal heroics are available for everyone, and painful times can be learned from and let go of.

I tried to explain this to my mother, but she couldn't see me as a hero. Rather, after a long pause, she found the most positive term to use to be *stamina*. Stamina that I have lasted so long.

I mentioned to a nursing friend of my mother that I had done a speech at a pharmaceutical company as a success story. She listened and then walked away without saying a word. She was a head nurse in the medical ward at the hospital who knew years ago about my condition. I have a lot of respect for her, but was left feeling awkward and shamed when she walked away.

When I am at work, I still go through mild cycles. If I'm fragile and I hear an air conditioner making a sound and find my mind correlating to it, I no longer respond with trepidation, but jump in to discover and enjoy any correlation with the sound and my thinking. It really changes the experience.

I am especially guarded about sleeping, as I can get into a bad state through lack of sleep and find it harder to sleep as a result. I'm careful to keep the stress level down.

I seem to be reclaiming the treasures of my past. I have a piano that was built in Toronto, dragged to the Rocky Mountains, where my mother grew up, brought to Montreal, where I grew up, and is now back in Toronto with me. I recently had the piano completely refurbished. It cost more than buying a new piano, but it means the world to me. It is solid oak and has the finest touch and sound of any piano I have played. I have recorded three new songs on it.

Along with the piano, I bought a Peugeot ten-speed bike off eBay. It is similar to the one I owned in the seventies, when I was in my teens. I lost track of it when I went to university. It just disappeared. Now it's back.

Recently I bought an MGB roadster sports car. It replaces the MGB I bought and lost track of. I have joined MG internet forums and find it very relaxing reading the many posts about all sort of esoteric mechanical trials and tribulations. I got a creeper for Christmas to crawl around under the car, ready to "fix" things.

I also have gotten very involved with chess, which I played in college. I am the youngest member of a chess/social club that has been going on for over fifty years. I also play online. I really enjoy playing, but when I am about to win, my hands start shaking, and I might scatter the board pieces. Losing poses no such anxiety.

As Joseph Campbell has put it: I am "participating joyfully in the sorrows of life."

So I continue my hero's journey, supported by my wife and family members with whom I have shared my story. I'm very proud of my son, who is at the beginning of his career and has proven to have gifts in personal relations with people. I greatly enjoy my extended family, including my wife's side. I look forward to being a grandfather. And I look forward to further adventures with my wife.

Community

If anyone would like to contact me I can be reached at email address cg.walker@ymail.com. I have also started an on-line forum: http://theoceanicmind.com for people with similar conditions to post their examples of synchronicity, energy work results and heroic events.

Bibliography

Chopra, Deepak. *The Path to Love.* New York: Random House Inc., 1997.

Jamison, K. R. *An Unquiet Mind.* New York: Alfred A. Knopf, 1995.

Maltz, Maxwell. *The New Psycho-Cybernetics.* New York: Prentice Hall Press, 2002.

Osborn, Diane K., ed. *Reflections on the Art of Living: A Joseph Campbell Companion.* New York: HarperCollins Publishers Inc., 1991.

www.ingramcontent.com/pod-product-compliance
Lightning Source LLC
Chambersburg PA
CBHW050545280326
41933CB00011B/1729

* 9 7 8 0 9 8 8 0 8 2 9 0 8 *